Military AND Mindful

# Advance Praise

"Benef reminds women that they are not alone and to seek support and community. She inspires them to acknowledge and savor their gifts, accomplishments and talents. To see their brilliance. She is authentic, relatable and sincere in her desire to help others. What a gift and service this book is to those who serve our country."

**Brahmani Liebman**, MSEd, RYT-500, Kripalu School of Yoga Faculty, co-director of Journey Into Yoga School of Yoga & Meditation.

"Ms. Verell is a very insightful, extremely capable young woman who is living what Zorba the Greek called "the Full Catastrophe"-- that is, life as a veteran, a spouse, a mother, engaged in an ambitious and meaningful career, and married to a spouse who gets repositioned on the globe every few years. Benef knows the challenges many of us face in our efforts to stay grounded, present and healthy while balancing many plates in the air. Listen to Benef! She is funny, wise and authentic and has a lot to teach us all."

**Robin Carnes**,
Co-Founder of Warriors at Ease, Author of "Sacred Circles: A Guide to Creating Your Own Women's Spirituality Group"

"LTC Verell shares practical perspectives and solutions that have not received enough emphasis in recent military personnel development courses. She is leading by demonstrating strength in vulnerability. Future military leaders will be more effective in the military and in life if they heed the lessons she had to learn from outside her military service."

**Timothy Avery**, PsyD,
U.S. Naval Academy Class of 2003

# Military
## AND
# Mindful

*Eight Essential Elements to*
*Manage Your Military*
*Career and Motherhood*

# Benefsheh Verell
Lieutenant Colonel, United States Army, Retired

NEW YORK

LONDON • NASHVILLE • MELBOURNE • VANCOUVER

# Military AND Mindful

Eight Essential Elements to Manage Your Military Career and Motherhood

Published in New York, New York, by Morgan James Publishing in partnership with Difference Press. Morgan James is a trademark of Morgan James, LLC. www.MorganJamesPublishing.com

ISBN 9781642794670 paperback
ISBN 9781642794687 eBook
ISBN 9781642795271 audiobook
Library of Congress Control Number: 2019901295

**Cover & Interior Design by:**
Christopher Kirk
www.GFSstudio.com

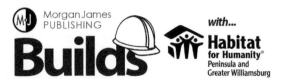

Morgan James is a proud partner of Habitat for Humanity Peninsula and Greater Williamsburg. Partners in building since 2006.

Get involved today! Visit
MorganJamesPublishing.com/giving-back

# Dedication

*For my children,
may you have the courage to acknowledge and
overcome your fears.*

*For all Service Members,
may you know that you are never alone.*

# Table of Contents

# Foreword

For me, the beginning of my spiritual, physical, emotional, mindfulness awakening came through pain. Enormous profound physical and emotional pain. They say you're in three states of a storm in life: Going into a storm, in the eye of a storm, or coming out of a storm. I was suffering and suffocating in overwhelming physical illnesses that kept getting worse day by day. I had two children and was pregnant with my third. My husband was constantly gone on TDY or deployment and my career was doing very well, in spite of my illnesses for years. I received a few great evaluations in a row from some awesome leaders that I enjoyed working for. But, through it all, I was hiding a gradual increase in pain and living a half life. I was driven to please anyone just for a pat on the back, and I allowed myself to get so busy with life in my roles wearing all the Super Woman hats that I lost my voice and what I needed most. I worked hard at work and worked hard at home. All the time, still never believing it was good enough. I spent countless Sundays in Mass praying for God to make me a better wife, a better mother, a better person. Then, I would trudge away day to day in this merry-go-round of tasks. I didn't realize it would take a toll on me eventually.

Surprising to me, I was still very successful in military terms, but something was happening. My body, mind, and soul grew restless and I couldn't figure out why. After my third child and a bout with numerous health issues, the next twelve months would change my life forever. I was rushed into emergency surgery while still on convalescent leave postpartum, but kept it close hold. I soon got promoted and had this image of a wonderful life and family others saw as perfect. All the time, I was hiding some near fatal diagnoses. For me, it was mind over matter. I had control over everything as long as I could perform at home and work. I tried to be Super Woman. I cleaned my home, cooked, cared for the children. My ego made it tough for some sweet babysitters to do their job, because I was so demanding. People always said, "I don't know how you do it all, especially without drinking coffee!" I took it as a compliment. In actuality, I was burning the candle at both ends and trying to be perfect. I am a busybody and a bit high strung, which the Army rewards. So, it was no surprise when I kept succeeding militarily, but my health and life were gradually falling apart.

One day during my lunch break, I stumbled across this small building and was curious about what it was. It was the wellness center on base. These two young ladies gave me a tour and showed me all the free services they had. I was still nursing and operating on little sleep with three kids now and a deployed spouse. They had a massage chair, nutrition classes, a full bod-pod for measuring body fat, and sleep analysis. I scheduled an appointment and learned I was truly operating like the walking dead. My sleep quality sucked, my weight was stagnant, and I wasn't fueling myself with enough calories to maintain work, life, and nursing demands. I was in the gym pushing myself harder, but no results. After looking at all elements of my wellness and receiving some support, my metabolism kicked back in and my sleep improved.

As I was feeling great about myself, life went well for a while. Then I became gradually nauseous every day and dizzy. I wasn't feeling like myself. The doctors tried a few things, but didn't do labs or take blood. I felt marginally well. Then, a few months later, I went into work and was injured in a freak accident and sustained a traumatic brain injury. I was admitted to the TBI clinic for treatment. Over the course of several weeks, I was put through tests and treatment. My body went into shock! My seemingly manageable pain in other areas were exacerbated by the TBI. I started having fainting spells, mini stroke-like symptoms at work and was med-evacuated to the hospital and admitted. I was practically living in the hospital. I lost feeling on the left side of my body for over a year, and acquired new symptoms on top of all the TBI issues: light sensitivity, vomiting, headaches, nausea, balance issues, etc. I had the added stress of a supervisor targeting me because I wouldn't lie for him. So as a form of retaliation, he refused to sign my leave for brain rest after my head injury.  For the first time in my life, I couldn't control everything. I felt helpless. I then had to do what one does when they hit rock bottom...pray! I did the one thing I knew how to do. I humbled myself and my ego and asked for help. My spouse came back in the midst of my first back procedure that went horribly wrong and caused shingles from the steroids they injected in my back and my own stress. He struggled with not knowing what to do to help me and became emotionally absent. I felt as though I was alone, but I kept praying. One day I turned on my radio and heard a famous pastor speaking about prayer and meditation. I had never given much thought to meditation, except occasionally in yoga. I realized I always prayed, which is our way to talk to God. I didn't realize meditation is God and the Universe speaking to and through us. I found all the answers to my most difficult issues were answered through meditation. I also found my prayers and mindset improved. I could relax my brain and just "Be". I started hearing positive words that started feeding my soul. As my soul found truth in these words day after day, I started to feel hope again. I began coping with my situation with walking meditations because it was all I could do physically. I was hunched over, dragging my left leg, but doing what I could between physical therapy and all my medical appointments. I was on a lot of medication and gradually weened myself off with yoga twice a week and regular meditation. I found a way to make it work for me by adding things to my life that I could physically do, like gardening. Then, my routine started manifesting positive outcomes and blessings beyond anything I could imagine.

Finally, my doctor called and said of thousands of candidates, I was chosen with six others to be a part of a special outpatient program called the Intense Outpatient Program (IOP) under the National Intrepid Center of Excellence (NICOE).

I was pulled out of my unit for a month and treated in a small group environment. I learned to incorporate pain management through yoga, stress management, mindfulness, sleep therapy, detoxification, alternative medicines, health, wellness, and so much more to bring a level of balance back into my life. They validated my pain was real and helped me cope and begin healing. Upon graduation, I had to incorporate the things I learned to suit my life and the career I still had. I was able to live a good life again. I was more mindful and could discern with my whole life before me, that in my greatest weakness, there was so much strength there. The pain made me dig deep and ask myself what I wanted out of life. I got my fire back through meditation and channeled it to deal finally with the supervisor that tried, but failed to ruin me. I went from wondering how I could go on living in so much physical pain, to how I would walk again, read again, and be able to run again for my children. I stopped defining myself by what I did for the military, but who I was in my core. Once my eyes were open and positive energy flowed to me, through me, and from me, I could give back the lessons and the answers to true freedom and joy. Once my ego got in agreement with my higher self and my soul's purpose, everything else came into union. My job was less stressful, my kids were my blessings and easier to be present for, my wants and needs were met. I can truly say my life was exponentially changed forever by what I learned in getting to this wonderful awakening of mindfulness and positivity. I incorporate waking from a place of gratefulness everyday to count my blessings. I am still serving our great country and utilizing what I am continuing to learn everyday. By no means have I "arrived", but I know, by the Grace of God, I have evolved to live my best life now. I can't tell you that life won't throw you a curve ball now and then. I won't tell you life will be perfect after you learn these techniques from this book.

But, what I offer you is the truth of how amazing these techniques can be if you fully embrace the concepts that Benef lays out in these chapters. If you allow yourself to let go and explore truth in yourself and just try to incorporate a little bit at a time, you will see a difference. It is all up to you. Everyone is different, so take your time and allow yourself to give back to you. This military life is great, but it's also one of the most stressful careers in the world. Add the nurturing and raising of a family and it is, by far, one of the most complex crucible experiences in life. The resiliency that comes from making these techniques a lifestyle will prove to be the best decision you've made for you, your career, and your family. We are abundant in our abilities to heal, grow, and love. Mindfulness is our link and gateway to a purposeful centered life.

Lesley G. Ortiz
Lieutenant Colonel, United States Army
Owner, L.W. Atelier Ltd. Co.

# Introduction

Being in the military is hard. That's a given. Whatever the reason we sign up, in the end we know that our service will require much sacrifice. If we've volunteered to serve when we're young and single, this may seem exciting and adventurous. The opportunity to travel the world, meet new people, and have new experiences attracts many of us who yearn for something more outside of our hometowns. We may deploy numerous times or the military may station us overseas, but the sense of freedom is still there even though we know we have a commitment and obligation to fulfill.

Then one day we have a family and everything changes. Now what was once difficult but adventurous and fun has become stressful and a source of constant anxiety. How do we manage to raise another human being (which we don't know how to do) and manage being in the military? Who will watch our baby when we have to go to the field or deploy? Where are we going to pump and how do we store the milk? How will we manage to get to PT at 0530 when the daycare doesn't open until 0600? What do we do when the daycare calls and says that our child has a fever and we have to come get him right away in the middle of the day? What will our coworkers think of us if we just up and leave or can't show up to work because our child is sick?

These are all valid questions and potential logistical nightmares that can make us feel guilty and as if we're failing at both being a mom and being in the military. The sense of guilt or shame we feel for not holding up our weight at work is real. The constant pulling in two directions between our child and work never seems to cease and we feel we must power through no matter the cost. We're military, after all. We understand adversity and working through problems. Isn't this just another problem that we must solve? Our partner is helpful, but has his or her own job to do that takes up just as much time and energy as ours. And, let's be honest, the mother usually ends up being the primary caretaker in most situations.

So where do we go from here? "Here" being the place of exhaustion, guilt, and a feeling that we must somehow balance being a mom and being in the military because we feel like we're failing miserably at both. One solution is to end our military service. This is a valid and decent solution that many of my classmates and coworkers opted to do. I admire them greatly, for they had the courage to take that leap of faith. But what if we do not have the courage or desire to leave the military? What if that isn't even an option for us due to a service commitment? Do we just continue to live in a state of anxiety and guilt about our perceived underperformance at work and our lack of quality time and mothering with our children?

The answer is no, we do not have to stay in this place of struggle and adversity. We can absolutely overcome our circumstances and learn to manage both being a mom and being in the military. We can have balance in our lives between our careers and our homelife. I realized that all this was possible (years after the fact) and that I did not have to struggle needlessly on my own in those early days of motherhood. After I retired from the Army, I gained a new sense of purpose in continuing to serve the military population. My mission became to help and mentor other women managing being a mom and being in the military. If I could perhaps aid another in her adversity or give her my knowledge before the struggle became overwhelming, this would be a great source of fulfillment to me.

This is the purpose of this book – to share my story and the success and failures I had as I managed being both a mother and service member. My hope is that by understanding where I screwed up, you can avoid those mistakes, and that by sharing how I eventually succeeded in finding a sustainable solution, you may get there quicker than I did. This is the goal of mentorship, after all. In the military we are taught to seek out and find mentors to guide us along our career. For whatever reason, I never had a mentor while in the Army. I certainly had my share of good leaders (and several bad), but no one that I felt was going through what I was going through with being a mom and being in the military. My peers, of course, were going through the same thing – that doesn't count as mentorship. We could barely make it to work on time, much less act as guides for each other. We didn't have the answers. The answers only come later upon having the seniority of age and experience. Then we could look back and say, "Ah yes, that is what I did wrong and this is how I should've done it."

In this book, I aim to give you those answers. This book is a reflection on twenty years of service, thirteen spent as dual military, and twelve spent as a mother. The mistakes are real, the pain is real. It hurts even to share some of them; I'm tearing up just thinking about it. But for you to trust me to lead you in your time of adversity, I must be vulnerable with you and not talk a bunch of crap. It was hard every single day. Had someone given me the tools and skills you will learn in this book about how to balance both being a mom and being in the military, I would've jumped for joy. So read on, dear one, and may this book give you the answers that you seek.

# CHAPTER 1

# Guilty at Home, Guilty at Work

As a dual military couple, my new husband, Thomas, and I started our marriage living in different locations. He, being four year groups ahead of me, was going through the Army's Intermediate Level Education at Fort Leavenworth, Kansas, while I was starting graduate school at the University of Maryland. I had chosen to accept a teaching position at the United States Military Academy and we both agreed that this was a good decision even though it meant being stationed in different places for about four and a half years. *We'll be fine*, we thought. We had been separated while we were dating and had overcome that situation, so this wouldn't really be all that different. As you know already, we were dead wrong.

My first child, Kamron, was born a little over a year after we were married. He was premature at thirty weeks and spent the next six weeks in the Neo-Natal Intensive Care Unit at what is now

Walter Reed Medical Center in Bethesda, Maryland. I had essentially two weeks off before school started, so that was all the maternity leave I had. Every day for six weeks, I went to the NICU and Thomas flew in every other weekend. The only saving grace during that time period was that my parents lived three miles from me and I had really close friends that also lived in the DC metro area. It was incredibly difficult coming home each night to an empty house, pumping every two hours, alone, with no husband and no baby. I binge watched a lot of TV and I made use, for the first time, of the counseling services that Military One Source offers. Basically, I was barely surviving.

As a geographically single mother, when the doctors finally let Kamron come home, I made extensive use of the "grandmother babysitting service." If you're lucky enough to have your parents in the area and they are able and willing to care for your child while you work, there is no better solution. I managed like this for the remaining year of grad school and then was off to West Point to spend three years as a professor teaching physical geography. The Army did its best and Thomas PCS'd to Fort Drum, New York, about a six-hour drive away. He would commute every weekend to be with us, but during the week, I was on my own.

It's lonely getting up each morning, preparing the milk and the bag for daycare. It hurt to have to drop Kamron off with a very nice stranger and then bravely face the unknown of my teaching job. West Point does a good job of preparing its new instructors with an intensive New Instructor Training course. It became apparent, however, that I had no idea what I was doing and was completely distracted during the day and during the evening when trying to prepare for the "practice-teach" sessions. My first practice lesson was on coastal geography. It went so poorly that they stopped it before the time was up and later my boss called me in to her office. I will say up front that everyone was very kind. This was a blessing that several of my peers did not have with their bosses. My boss said that she realized that I was going through things alone as a geographically single mother with no help at home. She said I needed a mother's helper or some kind of consistent daily help. She suggested I look into getting an au pair. I did this immediately. This was July and by October I had an au pair.

So on the surface, I had solved my problem of needing help. I still felt like a complete imposter at work, but that's probably a story for an entirely separate book. The routine became familiar, seeing Thomas on the weekends and barely keeping it together during the week. The au pair, Megan, turned out to be an amazing person and we had a great system where she helped in the mornings and evenings and also took Kamron to daycare so we could manage her hours efficiently for the times I needed the most help.

Somewhere along the way, Thomas and I decided we wanted a second child. We realized that if we waited for the Army to station us together, it would be several years before we had our second child and we didn't want such a huge age gap. Around the time that I became pregnant, the units at Fort Drum were going through rotations to Iraq. Thomas deployed for twelve months in the summer of 2007 and now I really was all alone. The weekends, which used to be a break for me, now became even harder than during the week. With my husband no longer available to shoulder the burden of child care, and Megan having weekends off, I was left to do everything for my son while also being pregnant and tired all the time.

I didn't enjoy teaching at all. Going to work was a burden and I felt like I wasn't giving my best. In fact, I knew I wasn't giving my best – I was sucking big time. I was too tired and didn't have any motivation to put the effort I needed into class prep to make my classes engaging or exciting. If any of my former cadets are reading this, I apologize for my crappy classes. My attitude at work was one thing, and my attitude at home was actually much worse. I was angry, I was unhappy, and it pissed me off that everyone around me seemed so happy. The neighborhood I lived in was like Mayberry. People were joyous and friendly. As disgruntled as I was, I did not want to see people happy. I wanted them to be miserable like me. I did not want to see happy families with fathers laughing and playing with their children. I felt as if a dark cloud hung over my head – and probably there really was one.

I remember being six or seven months pregnant, trying to give my squirming toddler a bath. I was on my knees and he wouldn't sit still. I was so tired and just wanted to sleep for three days straight. I hung my head and cried. I was never going to be out of this misery. I was all alone and drowning. There wasn't anyone that could help me and there was no one that understood what I was going through. How was I going to manage this? How was I going to make it through another day? When would this end? Clearly not anytime soon, as the Army extended my husband's unit to a fifteen-month deployment. I couldn't just quit. I still had two years left at this assignment and owed the Army another three years after that for my master's degree. Life sucked, without a doubt. I was in a dark place with seemingly no way out.

After the birth of my daughter, Violette, managing two kids on my own, as you would expect, did not get any easier. She didn't want to latch on for breastfeeding and that sent me into a depression spiral of my obvious incompetence at a simple motherhood task. I realized later that this isn't a simple task at all and that many people struggle, but since Kamron was too premature to breastfeed, I wanted so badly to get it right with this child. I was hard on myself, to be sure, saying unkind things to myself that I would never say to one of my Soldiers or friends. Day after day I told myself I was failing, incompetent, an imposter, and a really bad instructor. As you can imagine, this did nothing to improve my self-worth and my negative emotional state led to eventual physical illness. I had two bouts of bronchitis and laryngitis in one winter.

I honestly can't remember if I told my husband what I was going through at the time. I was able to talk to him on the class A line government phone in my office, but it wasn't daily and he was going through his own stuff. In the summer of 2008, when Violette was about three months old, things finally took a turn for the better. I'm not sure how I had found out about it, or why I decided to go, but I went to a weekend yoga retreat at the Omega Institute in Rhinebeck, New York. My mother came up to watch the kids and we had worked it out so that

Megan would also be with her the whole weekend. My only job was to try and enjoy myself and not worry about the kids.

That yoga retreat absolutely improved my mental and emotional states. In fact, just getting away and being by myself was a source of relief and inspiration. Upstate New York is incredibly beautiful in July and experiencing solitude in nature had such a healing quality that I didn't even fully recognize until years later. The most important aspect of that yoga retreat with famous yogi Seane Corn was that it sparked the idea that perhaps I could change things. There seemed the possibility of living without all this misery and guilt. I didn't know at the time how all this was going to be possible, but I felt a sense of peace and confidence that I had not felt in quite some time. I felt a sense of hope that things would get better and that I could be happy. I began to change the way I was thinking about things and I began to do yoga regularly.

I did not solve all my problems at that one yoga retreat, but I did realize that I had the power within me to solve my problems. I knew I could do it. I began to have the very beginnings of faith. Now, it would be some many years before I learned all the tools and skills I needed to navigate being a mom and being in the military. It would be almost ten years, right about the time I retired. Such is life.

Just like in the military, once we become experts at whatever job they've put us in, that is about the time we PCS and move to some other job in a new location and have to start all over again. There were many more ups and downs, as you may expect in the roller coaster of life. Clearly, I still had more to learn. However, the beginning, the spark, the first step out of the black hole began that July in 2008.

What follows in this book is the accumulation of what I learned over those ten years. The path that I had to walk to get there was bumpy and grossly unpleasant at times. I will share several of my stories, but some are just too personal to put in writing for the whole world to see. If, after reading this book, you decide to reach out to me, I guarantee you that if it pertains to helping you in some way, I will share my most personal stories. I want, after all, for you not to make the same mistakes that I have made. I want for you to be successful, confident, and strong. I want you to know that you can manage both being in the military and being a mom. You can do this without sacrificing your mental, emotional, and physical health. You can do this without feeling stressed out and guilty. You can be the leader you were meant to be in your service and be an amazing mother. Let me show you how.

CHAPTER 2

# The MINDFULL Way

Imagine for a moment that you are about to take a flight to a destination that you have never been to. Picture yourself waiting at the gate for the flight to board. You don't have a dedicated seat on this flight and are on standby. You've got to get on this flight, as it's the last one scheduled for the next several days and you want to meet your family whom you haven't seen for weeks. How do you think you would feel? Perhaps you may have some anxiety, nervousness, or fear about not making the flight. Your body may feel tense and your breath may be shallow. You keep thinking that if you miss this flight you're going to be so sad and disappointed, as you really miss your family. You pace back and forth and check the status board every two minutes. This is not an ideal situation at all.

Now imagine a vastly different scenario of how you'll be traveling on this flight. Now you are flying First-Class. You arrived at the airport and went to the VIP line at the counter and through security with no wait. You spend your remaining time in the club lounge relaxing while you wait for the flight to board. You are of course first to board the flight, get seated, and greeted by a friendly flight attendant who offers you the drink of your choice. You're feeling calm, excited to see your family, and confident that everything will go smoothly as you planned. You look forward to what will surely be a relaxing and enjoyable flight.

These are two very different scenarios. I'm betting the second option appeals more to you. What if I told you your life could be like the second option virtually all the time? You can feel like you're flying First-Class in your life. Would you want that for yourself? This book walks you through how to do exactly that the MINDFULL Way in the next eight chapters. If you follow the guidelines in these chapters, you can live a First-Class Lifestyle. You will see and experience the benefits in your physical, mental, and emotional health, plus be able to manage being in the military and being a mom.

Each chapter is a key element in the MIND-FULL Way, my program to aid you in figuring out how to manage your life without stress and guilt. They're ordered in such a way as to take care of practical matters first, but they don't necessarily have to be read in order. In Chapter 3, Manage Your

Resources, I talk about understanding balance and how to achieve it in your life as it pertains to work and family. Chapter 4, Increase Your Communication, discusses the ins and outs of communication and how to best communicate your needs to others so that you can be more efficient at work and at home. In Chapter 5, Navigate Your Emotions, I talk about feelings and discover what you can do to control your emotions so as not to lose your cool on the job or with your family. Chapter 6, Develop Your Mindset, is all about mindset and what you can do to stay on top of your game in any situation. Chapter 7, Find Your Power, focuses on power, and how to use your power in the most effective way to take care of your family while still excelling at work. In Chapter 8, Unleash Your Trust, I discuss how to build trust and why it's important to maintaining a First-Class Lifestyle. Chapter 9, Lighten Your Shadow, looks at possible obstacles that may pop up and how to overcome them. Chapter 10, Live and Maintain, discusses self-care and ways to continue practicing what you've learned.

It's taken me ten years to learn and understand all these elements of living a First-Class Lifestyle and put them into the MINDFULL Way for you. For sure I am still learning new things every day. One can never be done with the learning process, though one certainly can become an expert. Sometimes it takes us a few tries to learn one lesson, but eventually we get it. Just as we didn't master walking in one day, you probably won't master the lessons in this book in one day either. However, with continued focus and practice, you certainly can become an expert in managing your life and the skills it takes to successfully navigate being a mom and being in the military.

At the end of this book, you will have all the tools and skills I used to succeed in both my military career and at motherhood. I will say however that I did not do this alone. I hired coaches to help me along the way. I never would have learned half the stuff in this book without the help of a coach. They weren't military though and didn't have any affiliation with the military. I had to adapt the things they taught me so that they made sense in a military setting. Reading a book and then taking the action described in the book works quite well for a lot of people. Others, however, like to have people to support them. If you're a person who likes to have a cheerleader rooting you on, then please reach out to me. We can work together to develop and achieve your goals. My goal is to help you in the best way that I can, hence this book. Let's get started!

CHAPTER 3

# Manage Your Resources

I f we think back to that First-Class flight from the previous chapter, one thing is certain: When you travel First-Class, the airline staff makes sure you have everything you need to be comfortable and enjoy your flight. All of their resources are for your benefit and to make you feel relaxed and at ease. At work, your company, battalion, brigade, or the equivalent for your military branch has resources broken down into personnel/human, intelligence, training/operations, supplies/equipment, long range plans, and communications. This breakdown is so you can accomplish your mission efficiently and effectively. We feel satisfied at a job well done. But what about at home? Are you feeling like a First-Class passenger or standby? This could have something to do with how you're managing (or not managing) your resources. At home, the situation can model that of your work quite nicely with this familiar staff structure.

## Personnel – Build Your Team

First off, I do want to say that there really isn't any such thing as "balance" in life unless of course you are working with an actual dual scale. Balance by itself is a myth, I've found, and what we are really talking about is balance and counterbalance. There are times in your life when work will take precedence over family and vice versa. The trick is to become aware if it feels too weighted in any one direction and adjust accordingly. It's perfectly normal to feel like the people at work need you more in some circumstances than your family does. We're not indispensable to the people at work like we are to our family, and that is something to never forget. In the military especially, we are all replaceable. If we're not, the unit is doing something wrong. We can, however, implement strategies to make juggling family and work easier in our lives.

One important thing to remember is that we are never alone. Often, we choose not to ask people for help because we don't want to "burden" them. But how do we really know we are a burden if we never ask the person in the first place? By not asking, we've taken away the other person's decision to say yes or no. I understand that asking for help can be a touchy subject. I used to be against asking others for help, besides family, because that meant that I couldn't handle everything and that I did not have my stuff together, so I must be failing in some way. It was basically my ego and pride that prevented me from reaching out and caused quite a bit of unnecessary suffering. For the longest time, I refused to ask for help from the largest population available to me – the military spouses.

I do not fully understand how or why the "us vs. them" mentality developed between female service members and military spouses. It has got to be the most asinine nonsense I have encountered between a group of women, but I definitely felt it in my lieutenant and captain days. It must have been the ego and pride thing again. I honestly believed that these strong and resourceful women didn't do anything throughout the day except watch TV, nap, and drink sweet tea and margaritas. I soon learned that I was dead wrong. These women saved my sanity and came to my aid in my desperate time of need. It is precisely because they are working in the home that they could offer help with my children. They never hesitated to watch one of my children when they were sick, be my emergency contact, or cook meals for me when I was alone after the birth of my second child. Why had I been resistant to such generosity before? We are, after all, on the same team, the team of raising children that will grow up to become productive members of society. If you haven't already, it is essential that you reach out to this community, your community, and develop these relationships. The team you build at home is just as important as the team you build at work.

On the subject of working smarter at home, especially where both parents are military or have jobs outside the home, is outsourcing those tasks that just take up too much time. If both parents are working, then you can find the extra cash flow to hire someone to clean the house and do yard work or any chores that you do not enjoy. The hard-earned money that you are making deserves to go toward promoting your overall well-being. Hiring people to help you out even if only occasionally means you don't have to spend your precious down time doing chores and running around trying to get everything done. I'm a huge fan of outsourcing. After getting an au pair, I next hired a cleaning lady. For some, cleaning is almost meditative and helps them clear their minds – not so for me. What did make me feel relaxed and at ease was coming home to a house that was cleaned once a week.

We really don't have to do everything on our own. I don't know where we are taught this nonsense. Who says that we have to be perfect at everything in order to be a good mother or a good person? In most cases, we're lying to ourselves and suffering miserably for it. It's not easy to work and be a mother. It's also not easy to stay at home and be a mother. These women do not have it easier than we do. It's just as hard, albeit in a different way. Judging them for not working is just as insidious as people that judge us for working. There is no right or wrong answer on the matter. To work or not to work as a mother is an individual and family decision. I didn't have a choice but to keep working because I still owed a service commitment. However, many of my classmates chose to end their service once they had children. Some of them have regrets and some don't. My point is that neither choice is wrong. It's a choice we make given the knowledge we have at the time.

If you haven't been prone to ask for help from others before, then this may not be an easy concept to accept right off the bat. One tool that has been very useful to me is to genuinely acknowledge all my accomplishments. Get out a piece of paper and list all your accomplishments while serving in the military. These may be things that would go on an evaluation report, but also, those tasks you've done or people you've helped that cannot be captured in your evaluation report because they are not quantifiable to the military. Perhaps you helped a fellow co-worker through a divorce, addiction, or trauma. Maybe you volunteer regularly or have worked behind the scenes to help your spouse achieve his or her career or personal goals. Handwrite everything that you have done and don't be afraid to put the littlest things on the paper. Often as women we tend to downplay our accomplishments, gifts, and talents. I can only speak for myself as to the reason, but I tended to think the things I've done weren't a big deal and that anyone else could do them just as easily. Your accomplishments are, however, a very big deal, and not everyone has done exactly what you have done. You need to own your worth and acknowledge your value. Once you can physically see on paper all that you have actually done, you can gain some perspective on your current situation of feeling stressed and overwhelmed. You're already a superhero and even superheroes team up to become even stronger and accomplish more together. I like to think of The Avengers with myself in the role of Captain America (he was in the military, after all!).

Next, take another piece of paper and write down a list of people who you think could offer support. These could be family members that live close by or spouses in the neighborhood or your friends. Determine how you think each person could help you in some way. You don't want to tap the same person too many times, so it's best to have a few different people from which to choose. Who might be able to pick up a child from daycare or school? Which responsible teen could watch your dog or water your plants for a small fee while you're gone? Who can be on your list of babysitters so you and your spouse or partner can have a night off or so that you can go get a massage or just grocery shop by yourself? The people are out there. It's the physically asking them to help us that is the hardest part. This takes practice and may feel awkward at first. If it does feel weird, then start small – maybe borrow a lawn mower or an iron. Or, don't ask for anything at all right away and just chat. Honestly, it took me about four more years before I really started asking neighbors for help. Our next duty station was in Virginia and I was once again near the safe haven of family. It took moving across the world to Korea for me to come out of my shell as the family option was definitely gone. Will asking for help require some reciprocity on your part? Most likely. We're building relationships here, not taking advantage of people. Unless you're paying someone, at some point you may be asked to repay the favor. For me that meant becoming involved in Family Readiness Group activities and helping with events the best I could. I couldn't always reciprocate the exact favor, but being present and visible showed that I cared and valued the help I received and the eventual friendships I made. However, you know this is what it means to be part of a team. It's no different than organizing and managing your team at work. Every person has a role and those tasks that he or she does best. The difference at home is that the people are not assigned to work with you. You have to physically ask them, which means letting go of your ego.

The final tool to building your team is to make a list of those chores or tasks that you do not enjoy doing so that you can outsource them. I'm talking about cleaning, cooking, laundry, yard work, whatever it may be for you. You have money – use it for your benefit, especially if your partner is deployed or working long hours.

So now we understand that asking for help is actually the brave course of action and what resilient people do to move forward. They use the resources that are available to them. We can stay stuck trying to do everything ourselves, or we can reach out and ask for help when we need it. It is not an easy thing to do, I know. The alternative, however, is to remain exactly where we are, which we've already identified as being unpleasant.

### Intelligence – Mindfulness Practices

Okay so mindfulness practices don't exactly correlate to what we think of as intelligence, but since I'm modeling off of a typical unit staff structure, I felt mindfulness worked best here for this breakdown of resources. What follows next is how to get our act together when it comes to how we manage work when we're at work and home when we're at home. If you have the type of job that allows you to leave work matters at work, then that is a huge blessing. Often, however, we bring all that crap home in the form of either emotional baggage or actual work that has to be done. This could be papers to grade (as was my case at West Point) or perhaps you're in a leadership position and are getting calls or emails at all hours of the day. The bleed over from work into personal life is a real problem and disrupts any type of tranquility we wish to experience in our family and home life.

Now, to be honest, if you're a commander or first sergeant, work is likely to follow you home. You do have the knowledge of knowing that it's not permanent and you will eventually rotate out. Being in a critical leadership position falls into one of those categories where the people at work often do need you as much as the family at home. But how do we compartmentalize? Is that even something we want to do? I often found myself worrying about my children while I was at work. That seems like a perfectly normal thing to do, but it left me distracted and wishing the work day was over. I would miss critical information in meetings because my mind simply wasn't there. Never mind that a lot of the meetings were boring. Then, while at home, I would find myself worrying about class preparation or a presentation that I had to do and not focusing on feeding or playing with my children. Again, my mind was somewhere else besides the present moment.

So how do we keep the mind from wandering off into some other activity? Is that even really possible? How do we prevent ourselves from worrying about the future or having anxiety about some upcoming event? It takes much practice and much discipline to train the mind. Think back to your first PT test, the initial test you had to take upon entering basic training. If you were like me, it probably sucked and was extremely difficult. Or maybe you were already in great shape and you did really well. The point is that after the several weeks of physical training, your scores on the PT test at the end of training improved, probably drastically. Increasing your physical fitness takes discipline, practice, and time. The same is true for improving your mental fitness and learning to be present in the moment.

The best way to bring the body and mind together in the present moment is through meditation. Before you stop reading and throw the book away, let me demystify meditation. Meditation is *not* emptying your mind of all thoughts. It does not have to be about sitting cross-legged in silence for hours. It is not about any religion, but can become a spiritual practice. You don't have to do any chanting or listen to anything that makes you feel uncomfortable in any way. Meditation is very personal and there are multiple ways to do it. No one way is correct or incorrect. Meditation is simply about being in the present moment with your mind, body, and breath.

## Meditation Focusing on the Breath

An easy way to meditate is to concentrate on the breath. The breath is one thing we can control, especially in times of crisis or stress. In fact, we are taught breath control during weapons training. If you want a steady shot, you've got to control your breath. This is mindfulness! The same principle applies to all other situations. If you want to be calm and present of mind, steady your breath. We can bring our attention to our breath and control our inhales and exhales. One method is to inhale for four counts, hold for four, exhale for four counts, hold for four, and then repeat for as long as you like. When you make the exhales equal or greater in count to the inhales, you begin to activate the parasympathetic nervous system and can calm the body and mind down in as little as two or three minutes. The nervous system is made up of two parts, sympathetic (fight or flight) and para-sympathetic (which is responsible for calming and relaxing the body, rest and digest). Your mind has to be focused on your breath in order to continue to breathe in this manner, exhales longer than inhales. Since breathing is something our bodies do automatically, when we focus our mind on the breath, we are in the present moment. When you notice your mind has wandered to some thought (which is completely normal and expected), you can gently bring your attention back to the breath. In this way, you teach yourself to be present in the moment and also aware of your thoughts. You can set a timer for as little as one or two minutes and this counts as meditation. If you're new to the idea of meditation, doing this once or twice a day is a great place to start.

## Meditation on Sight and Sound

Meditation is about keeping the mind focused on one thing at a time. If concentrating on the breath does not appeal to you, you can choose an image to look at, or repeat a meaningful word in your head (love, peace, joy, etc.) over and over again. It may just be me, but I find the drone of a C-130 sooth-ing (and ominous) and would go out walking in the cool night air on the base in Balad, Iraq just to hear them. The sound could be the ocean, the hum of a tracked vehicle, rain falling, it doesn't matter as long as it allows your mind to focus on that one entity. Each time you notice your mind thinking, bring your attention back to the sound, image, or the word. There are several free guided meditations available on apps like Insight Timer. I love guided meditations because the facilitator will remind me to concentrate and focus. I teach yoga and meditation and have my own personal practice, but I always benefit from working with an experienced teacher. The best way to learn to meditate is through continued experiential practice. Expect to have to start over repeatedly. The mind is like an untrained puppy. It'll be distracted by everything. We would treat a puppy kindly as we're trying to train it. The same is true of your mind.

## Meditation with Movement

Often there are times when I do not want to sit still at all. This is when I do a walking meditation or attend a yoga class. However, any type of repetitive movement can be a meditation as long as the mind is focused on that one activity. For walking, you would focus on how it feels to place one foot in front of the other, the sensations in the feet and legs as they move. The mind is focused on the sensation of walking. You can do the same while running. When you notice a thought, you bring the mind back to noticing sensation in the body. This concept applies to doing dishes, gardening, biking, swimming, any activity where your mind can focus only on the sensations in the body associated with that movement. Many physical activities can serve as a form a meditation. However, I'll note that focusing on sensation in the body may not be the best idea when doing extreme physical activities such as long road marches, but you'll have to determine what works best for you.

Using meditation to train the mind to focus on one task helps you in time to improve focus at work and focus at home. Meditation will help you to observe your thoughts and if they've wandered, to bring them back to what you are doing whether at home or at work. The ability to multitask is also another myth, like finding balance. The conscious brain cannot multitask. It just ends up doing neither task all that well. Have you tried to talk on the phone while your child is also trying to talk to you? I usually end up hearing parts of both conversations, but missing the point of each entirely. My vice is trying to look at Facebook while my daughter is trying to talk to me. I cannot read and listen well at the same time. There isn't any reason to try to do both things at once. This is how people misplace items, run into things, or forget things, because they were trying to multitask. Ever leave behind a weapon or other sensitive item? I have, and you can bet my mind wasn't present when I left those night vision goggles in the dirt. We already know about trying to talk on the phone (or text) and drive at the same time. It doesn't work and is dangerous. To work optimally, the mind must focus on one thing at a time and can then work faster so you can move on to the next task.

## Training and Operations – Time Management and Organization

Identifying how to work smarter at home with a team will help you manage your time more efficiently and organize your life more effectively. I am the queen of calendars and schedules (sometimes to a fault). Over the years I've developed and honed my systems and you will have to develop a system that works for you. I like to see things written down in front of me so I use actual paper calendars and schedulers. This also comes from years of working in a SCIF (Sensitive Compartmentalized Information Facility) where I couldn't bring my phone into the building or to any meetings. So, I took to maintaining a calendar that I carried with me and a white board calendar at home, each color-coded by family member. It's anal, but it's what I need. I won't remember anything if I don't write it down or make some sort of list.

Figure out what works for you and start using it. If you are a brand-new mom, it's tough to suddenly have another person to care for as well as yourself. Maybe you are lucky and your spouse manages the household calendar and you just have to refer to it, but often the primary caregiver is also the person who manages the family schedule. The schedules will only grow more complicated as the children get older and have more activities. Establishing a system early on will help greatly for your peace of mind. Like I said, I am a master at time management and organization. I can help you with this. I planned my entire wedding while working full time and my boss had no idea. And yes, I was planning while I was at work and exceeding the standards for getting all my work done. For years, I chose to downplay my talents and claim that I really never had that much work to do or that my job wasn't as difficult, and that was how I was so organized and efficient. My husband finally called me out on this and continues to call me out when I try to downplay my talents. You too have talents and skills. When they come naturally to us, we tend not to notice them as anything extraordinary. We may not have even identified them. It wasn't until I met one of my mentors, Meredith, that I understood the importance of identifying my brilliance and how to even go about doing that. A simple formula looks like this: Your Brilliance = it's really easy for you + people compliment you or wish they could do it like you. It will take some self-reflection or you can ask a close friend to help you. Once you identify your brilliance, you can then determine how to best use your talent to your advantage as you navigate being a mom and being in the military.

One thing I need to make clear: you may have the best organization system in the world, but if there are too many things on your plate, you won't get all of them done. This is a lesson I had to learn the hard way, twice. When I PCS'd I'd sign myself up for numerous activities to get involved in the community. I'd teach yoga, take dance classes, teach Sunday School, participate in the spouse club, and, oh by the way, the kids had their activities and I was still working full time. There aren't enough hours in the day to do all these things if we have to spend about a third of the time sleeping and another third or so at work. The solution? Exactly the same as if at work: prioritize, prioritize, prioritize. You may want to do everything because you have the best intentions to help others or it sounds fun, but the hard reality is you can't do everything. It's very embarrassing to have to renege on something you've promised. I became so overwhelmed that I had to stop everything because I got sick and was just too tired. Sorry, I can't teach yoga anymore and I know there's no other instructors. Sorry, I can't take dance anymore and I know this will mess up the formation for the recital. Sorry, I can't teach Sunday School anymore, but I'm too exhausted to go to church anyway. Sorry, yeah forget it, not doing the spouse club thing. I wasn't exercising at all. I could only barely manage going to work and coming home to throw something together for dinner. Clearly my brilliant time management and organization skills were falling flat without the ability to prioritize. I've since developed an acronym, SAGE, to assist with prioritizing and I discuss it in depth in the Develop Your Mindset chapter.

Taking care of your body also falls into this category by eating healthily and exercising. This is common sense, but often we just neglect to prioritize our exercise and food until it becomes critical. While at West Point, I used to long for the days of organized unit PT, because then I would get it done. PT on my own meant no PT until like a month before the PT test. In later units, I had to juggle getting the kids to daycare by 0530 or find a babysitter to come to the house, but I was exercising. One of my fellow instructors at West Point introduced me to what he called the "Tripod" method of determining a person's disposition. Imagine a three-legged stool. Each leg represents a gauge. The first is for hunger, the second is for fatigue, and the third is for temperature. If you skip breakfast in your rush out the door, by mid-morning you're likely famished. You've just taken out the hunger leg and are teetering on the two remaining legs. If you were up all night with a sick and vomiting child (why is it always chunks?), you're certainly exhausted by now as well and a second leg goes down. You've now crashed and burned. Though you couldn't have avoided staying up all night, you know you need to eat and could've kept two of the three legs working. This concept works exceptionally well for children. Snacks, naps, and wraps to keep them fed, rested, and warm (or unwrapped to keep cool).

## Equipment and Supplies – Shopping for Everything and Your Budget

What I'm talking about here is the way you go about getting the things you need for yourself and to make your household run smoothly. Grocery shopping used to be the bane of my existence. I didn't have time to shop every day, but going once a week meant that the fresh fruits and vegetables usually ended up going bad before I had a chance to use them. The services that deliver groceries to your house didn't exist when I lived off base and that wasn't an option overseas, so shopping became a chore I despised. The solution changed as my situation changed but involved Thomas and I sharing the task and sometimes eating out. You may be okay with grocery shopping, it may be your chance to get away. Perhaps it is clothes shopping that stresses you out. During my four years as a cadet in the fashion black hole that is West Point, I lost all ability to put together an outfit and never really regained the skill. At school and in the Army, I was wearing a uniform every day and not going anywhere at night. What did it matter? Occasionally, I might go out on the weekend; jeans and a nice top were fine. But, what you wear can actually have an impact on how you feel. Would you feel squared away if your uniform was not? When I started wearing Winnie the Pooh t-shirts and matching plaid shorts to neighborhood barbecues, my friend Shay staged an intervention. I recognized that I'd lost my mojo in the fashion area. I still don't like shopping. That's why there are personal stylists and Stitch Fix. The basic rule of thumb here is if it stresses you out or makes you feel bad, then you've got to find someone to help you, whether it's groceries, clothes, car maintenance, computers, or whatever else.

The family budget is also something that changes drastically when adding new family members. Unlike calendars and schedules, budgeting is not one of my strengths and I did seek outside help for this. It's important to know what income is coming in versus what you're spending each month. This is pretty standard stuff, but deserves mentioning in that it is yet another task you have to be aware of and manage.

## Long Range Plans – Vacations/Time Off

If you want time off, you have to plan for it. It's challenging trying to match up schedules (kids, spouse, work), but it's not impossible. You need the vacation and so does your family. I talk more about it in the Live and Maintain chapter, but recognize that scheduled time off is a necessity.

## Communications – Self and with Others

The whole next chapter covers this very important element. Many books exist on the subject. If you've ever had comms go down during the middle of an operation or exercise, then you know what it's like to be royally screwed. It's the same at home. If you and your partner, or you and your kids, aren't communicating effectively, then FUBAR operations have begun.

Remember that you do not have to try and do everything all at once and by yourself. You wouldn't (and shouldn't) do this at work, so why do this at home? Using your time wisely and efficiently means building a team and organizing your resources so you can accomplish everything you need and want to do. Following the suggestions in this chapter will help you do just that. Putting the systems in place to help you run things smoothly will allow you to feel like you would flying in First-Class – relaxed and confident. You are not alone. I am here to help you and there are at least a dozen other people you can ask for help. Sure, some of them may say no, but that's the worst they can do: say no. More likely they will be more than willing to help or will know someone else that can help you. And for those tasks that you can pay someone else to do, there's no reason to delay. Your mental, emotional, and physical well-being are worth the cost to hire someone to assist you. Asking for help is a sign that you understand your limits and are courageous in your desire to take the best care of yourself and your family.

CHAPTER 4

# Increase Communications

*"The relationship you have with yourself
is the most important relationship
in your life."*
– *Taming Your Outer Child*, Susan Anderson

It's about midway through your First-Class flight and you become thirsty. You press the call button and when the flight attendant comes, you ask for water. In that simple act you've communicated your needs to another person. Two things happened, you knew what you needed and the flight attendant was actively listening to you. The two key factors in communicating are being clear on what you need and being present and actively listening to those with whom you communicate.

## Show Up for Yourself First

This is all about self-communication. How do we determine what it is that we need and want?

We ask ourselves. This seemed silly to me when I first started to do this. Of course I know what I need, don't I? Well no, not really. What I knew was what I thought was expected of me and what I thought others wanted me to do. I had never sat down and asked myself what I needed and wanted, much less taken the time to really ponder and write my thoughts down. But how can you communicate your needs to others if you don't even really know them yourself?

There are a couple of really good exercises to get at the heart of what it is you really need and what you want, which are two very different things. Needs are those things you must have to survive physically, mentally, and emotionally (google Maslow's hierarchy of needs). Wants and desires are those things that aren't absolutely necessary, but would make life that much sweeter and are icing on the cake (cake being your needs). Susan Anderson in her book *Taming Your Outer Child* suggests a self-dialogue exercise in which your adult self asks questions of your inner child (around the age of five). You respond as a child would, using short and simple sentences. You can even write in your non-dominant hand. The purpose is to cut through all the crap we tell ourselves about should, could, and would and get to the real heart of what it is we need or desire. For example, when I did this exercise myself on the topic of physical activity and working out, I spent two minutes getting quiet and concentrating on my breath and then I asked little me, "We need to work out more. What do you want to do for exercise?" She said *"I want to dance and play. You never let me dance. We always have to run or go to the gym. I hate running. I hate the gym. It's boring. I want to dance."* "But little, we have to run. We have to take the PT test, and to do well, we need to run. But, I will turn the music on and we will dance and have fun." This is one way to communicate your needs to yourself. I'm happier when I take the time and allow myself to dance. There are things that you need to do for yourself to be content and fulfilled and you have to figure out what they are.

Another self-communication exercise I like to do is journaling. Now if you don't like to write, just hear me out. I used to think journaling meant writing everything I was thinking out in a notebook and I would do this for what seemed like ages and pages at a time. This is one method, but it's time consuming and I would go for days or weeks without writing. Another and more productive method of journaling comes from Julia Cameron's book *The Artist's Way: A Spiritual Path to Higher Creativity.* She recommends what she calls "The Morning Pages." It's three pages of writing first thing in the morning. You write whatever you want for three pages, no more, no less. The three-page limit makes it manageable and the fact that you are writing daily makes it consistent. Over time, you'll see your needs and wants show up on the pages in the form of complaints, judgments, or questions. You have to show up for and take care of yourself first before you can communicate with or take care of others. We often do not do this and wonder why we're exhausted, irritated, and unhappy. Write the morning pages and they will tell you exactly why.

## Communication with Coworkers vs. Your Partner

The most important tool I've learned in communicating effectively with others is the art of active listening. Unfortunately, I didn't realize this or know how to do it until I'd taken my yoga teacher training in 2012. Prior to that, I was a terrible listener. My mind wandered frequently, often at my own choosing. If I perceived that a person was boring me (I'd make this assessment within the first thirty seconds), I would stop listening completely and think about something else. Occasionally, I would pop back in to see if the person had decided to say anything interesting and then go off into my own world again. Can you imagine how this must have come across to the other person? Whether or not they can actually tell if I'm listening, subconsciously people are aware and it's a huge turn off, even if they don't know why they are turned off. It's also just plain rude and arrogant. But our minds wander, whether by choice or because we cannot control it. The mindfulness exercises in the previous chapter are invaluable to increase your active listening skills. Being fully present in the moment and aware of your own thoughts and emotions is essential to communicating effectively with other people. If we want to get our needs across to our partner, family, friends, and coworkers, we have to be able to listen fully and know in the first place what it is that we need and want.

At work, I felt comfortable in my leadership role, being in charge, giving orders, and delegating tasks. There is nothing wrong with this and this was exactly how I needed to communicate with the people at work. Then when I went home as a geographically single mother with a live-in au pair, a toddler, and a baby, I was very much still the one in charge, giving orders, and delegating tasks. When Thomas came home on the weekends, he didn't want to disrupt the routine, being there for less than forty-eight hours, and things went relatively smoothly.

But what do you think happened when we were finally living in the same house after spending four and half years apart? Let's just say the reintegration did not go as I had envisioned. Looking back, I see now that I took on more responsibility at home than I should have, essentially pushing him out. He then did less because I was allowing him to do less. I began to think he wasn't competent and he began to feel he wasn't competent. What a mess and the perfect situation to create resentment between two people. Fortunately, I deployed, which forced a role reversal that proved Thomas was capable and competent in taking care of the household and the children. But what was really going on? I was so used to being in charge that I had forgotten how to work as a team with my partner. I had my team at work that I was responsible for leading and my team of supporters at home that I was responsible for leading and because my husband was living somewhere else and deployed, I simply wasn't used to having him around. When we finally lived together, I subconsciously treated him as a team member instead of an equal and co-leader. I didn't ask for his opinion in making decisions or consider his needs. I refused to give up or let go of the reins. This is not good for a partnership and our marriage paid the price at the time.

So how can you do this better and avoid the mistakes that I made? Communication is the answer of course, but not just any type of communication. Your yelling at your partner that he or she is lazy and not helping you will not make the situation any better. As I said earlier, effective communication starts with active listening. You've already identified what you need and want from the journaling exercises I've suggested. Now it's time to find out what your partner needs and wants. You have to ask and then be willing to listen without interrupting. It's so hard, I know. I so badly want to add my two cents in and explain myself. This is not the time. What your partner says may not be an accurate account of what you think and feel, but the point is just to let him or her talk and answer the question that you have asked. I've also missed a great deal of conversations because I was thinking about what I was going to say next instead of listening to what the person is actually saying. How many times have you not remembered the name of someone you've just met? It's usually because you were thinking about how you were going to introduce yourself rather than listening to the person say his or her name. It's embarrassing and the opposite of being present. The mindfulness practices in the previous chapter will help you to stop doing this.

Once your partner has finished talking, then you can restate what you heard in your words to validate that you were listening. People really want to know that they have been heard. I do not claim to be a couple's counselor, but listening to your partner (without judgment if you can) is extremely important.

Then hopefully you can begin a dialogue of give and take and mutual agreement, for you are co-leading the same team, not in competition with one another. These conversations can be extremely difficult and uncomfortable. However, if you let fear or guilt be the basis for your decision to not have a conversation, it never bodes well. I talk more about this in the Develop Your Mindset chapter. Dozens of books have been written on effective communication. I've barely scratched the surface, but have shared the highlights of what worked for me. Learning to communicate is a continuous and iterative process, as the conditions are constantly changing. It requires much self-awareness and a willingness to grow as an individual (and as a couple) if you want to get better at communicating with others. In my yoga teacher training class, I learned to use the acronym THINK when speaking with others. Is it True, Helpful, Inspiring, Necessary, and Kind? If you can answer "yes" to all five of these questions, then whatever you want to say is worth communicating. This works well for conversations that may seem confrontational, especially with coworkers, and also for speaking with children. I've stopped myself many times from speaking because my thought was either dripping in sarcasm (not helpful or inspiring) or some sort of gossip (probably not true, definitely not necessary), both of which are not kind. I'm not perfect, but I am aware, which means that I can stop unkind, passive-aggressive, or angry dialogue, whether internal or external, much quicker now.

# CHAPTER 5

# Navigate Your Emotions

*"Biography Becomes Biology"*
*– Anatomy of the Spirit,* Caroline Myss, Ph.D.

Emotions. They straight up suck – the "bad ones," that is. No matter what class you're flying, you'll have to deal with occasional turbulence, and emotions can be very turbulent. I've been in dark places, trapped with rage, jealousy, and despair. There seemed to be no end to my pain, and truth be told I often wanted to be there. It somehow felt comfortable "knowing" that I was inadequate, unlovable, and worthless. I "knew" that the world would somehow be better off without me. I never contemplated taking my own life, but I definitely thought to myself, "If I were to get hit with a stray bullet right now, well, that would be okay." No. That is definitely not okay. These thoughts are not healthy, but they come nonetheless. I didn't know in those days that I had a choice

I could make about these thoughts. Thoughts and emotions are so closely related, it's difficult to separate the two. With this chapter, I'll tackle emotions and how they connect with thoughts and then get more into how thoughts work with mindset in the next chapter. Understanding the choices you have when it comes to your emotions and thoughts is essential to living a First-Class Lifestyle. They can hold you hostage otherwise in a never-ending cycle of fear and terror, just as if you were a hostage on an actual plane. However, as uncomfortable as these subjects can sometimes be, this is where the real personal growth happens.

Let's dive right in to the subject of your emotions. I often found that expressing how I really felt about myself, another person, or a subject at work could only happen on rare occasions. I usually didn't want to experience the pain of being honest with myself or other people. It's easier to not confront a person (or yourself) than to think that you've hurt his or her feelings. However, being a leader in the military, I had to find a kinder and more constructive way to tell a person I thought he was underperforming (rather than "you're an idiot") or risk the mission not getting accomplished. I had to go hole up in the bathroom when I felt tears of frustration and anger about to erupt like a long overdue volcano or risk appearing out of control and overly emotional. In short, we sometimes have to hide our true feelings at work or at home to either save us from embarrassment or prevent us from straight up being mean. How then, and when, do we express and release these emotions in a constructive manner?

First, understand that you are perfectly normal for feeling sad, angry, jealous, frustrated, or irritated at work and at home. You are allowed to feel these emotions just as you are allowed to feel happy, excited, proud, love, or those emotions that you consider to be "positive." When we don't allow ourselves to feel emotions or think we shouldn't feel a certain way, we either stuff them down or bottle them up. Neither one of these options is good for your mental or physical health, and generally they result in us eventually acting out with less-than-desired behavior.

## Feelings from the Past

The first time I heard anything about energy anatomy was at the yoga retreat with Seane Corn back in 2008. The idea that emotions from previous events in my life could become trapped in my body and manifest themselves as disease or physical illness was mind-blowing. The thought of every past lover having left an energetic imprint in my body was not in the least appealing. How much yoga did

I need to do to get these dudes out of my system? Gross. I got my hands on any reading material I could that dealt with energy anatomy. The subject came up again in my yoga teacher training at the Kripalu Institute. We learned that our physical body is just one part of our system. We also have an energetic body.

The mind and body are not separate entities working independently of each other. Through my yoga teacher training and continued yoga training with Warriors at Ease, I learned that all events in our lives, especially the significant ones, come with an emotional charge that then becomes stored in the body. The emotion is especially powerful for those that have experienced trauma.

My Warriors at Ease instructors explained the science of what actually is happening in our brains and bodies during traumatic, stressful, or very emotional events. When we're experiencing these events, our amygdala sounds the alarm in the body, pumping out cortisol and putting us in fight or flight mode. The thinking brain, the pre-frontal cortex, essentially goes offline as a result of these stress hormones and we operate under the reptilian brain, our instinct for survival mode. The amygdala assigns an emotion to that experience, but because the thinking brain is offline, the body stores the memory as sensory data (sight, sound, taste, touch, smell). This becomes "the issues in the tissues" where we may feel chronic pain, inflammation, tension, headaches, or any other number of ailments, illnesses, or diseases. These stress chemicals need a way to be released or dumped so that the body can resume normal operations. Often, our pre-frontal cortex (thinking brain), prevents the chemicals/hormones from being released because we continue to revisit the event and think about the stressful situation over and over. Or our thinking brain rationalizes the event away, however the sensory data still remains in our body. Our energy goes essentially where our thoughts take us. If we're continuously thinking about a time in the past when someone harmed us, then our energy is going into the past. This is why we need movement and exercise, to discharge all this excess energy and the chemicals that we no longer need after an event has passed.

Those in the yoga community understand this mind-body connection and that emotions, if not processed, can become trapped in the body. Yoga, which facilitates being present with the mind, body, and breath through a series of postures and meditation, can release emotions that remain in the body. I've taught many yoga classes where people just start crying for no apparent reason as emotions come to the surface and release. In my personal yoga practice, I've experienced intense emotions many times while in a posture. One example I will share occurred about eight or nine years ago while I was in a reclined restorative posture. After several minutes of being in the posture, focusing on my breath and sensation in the body, I noticed a localized dull, but strong, pain in my right lower back. I began to focus on that point and "drop-in" and become aware only of that pain. At some point, the image of a man popped into my head. This was the man who molested me when I was five or six years old. Interestingly, I felt only detached compassion for this individual. It occurred to me that for someone to harm a child, he or she must be in a horrible dark place of self-hatred and misery. I was able to forgive my molester in that moment and the pain began to dissipate. I then continued on with my practice.

What I described above was my first experience with how emotions from past events release themselves from within the body. Yoga is how I choose to release these emotions and, because there are so many different types of yoga, I recommend a yoga practice for everyone. There really is a yoga class for every "body." I've taught yoga to people with missing limbs, those with back and hip issues, people with traumatic brain injuries, and those with severe PTSD or military sexual trauma. You do not have to have any pre-existing level of flexibility and you never have to look like the yogis on the cover of Yoga Journal. If all you do is lay down and concentrate on your breath for the whole class, you are still doing yoga and meditation.

I've had several of my yoga students come up to me and explain that over the course of a few weeks, not only had their physical pain or tightness start to dissipate, but mentally their heads felt clearer as well. Though they may not have consciously realized it, the yoga was helping them to release pent up tensions and body memories.

## Feelings in the Present

Yoga, along with meditation, is a practice for learning to be present in the moment with our mind and body exactly as they are. We can learn to observe our thoughts and notice if we are comparing or judging ourselves in any way and then accept who we are and how we show up in that moment, understanding that we are constantly changing and evolving. How we are today is not the same as how we were yesterday or how we will be tomorrow. Today I may feel pain in my lower back that I didn't have yesterday, or notice that I am sad or angry. Through repeated observation of our thoughts and feelings with yoga and meditation, we begin to notice how fluid thoughts and emotions are and that we are not only our thoughts and emotions. We can detach from a thought or emotion and observe it as a compassionate witness. This healthy form of detachment eventually allows us to feel and move through emotions much quicker than if we were to continue to fixate on them and the thought that we associate with the emotion.

The unthinkable happened to a friend of mine. Her baby died. She put the child down for a nap and a few hours later when she came to check, the baby was no longer breathing. There are no words of comfort. When I found out about this, there was nothing I could think of to say. As she was expressing her pain, I felt pain as a mother and I could empathize. The only thing I could tell her to do was to take each breath one at a time and essentially live from moment to moment. You cannot escape that kind of pain and horror. I could not tell her to "work through it." That is not my place, nor is it helpful in the least. I did help her, however, to focus and concentrate on one breath at a time. For in that one breath, that one moment, she was present with the pain and moving forward at the same time. That one breath eventually turned into a few seconds, a few minutes, an hour, a day. There is no set time for experiencing grief. We can only be present, moving forward one breath at a time.

Recognizing that your emotions are a primary factor in how you operate in daily life is a huge step toward awareness and allowing yourself to acknowledge them. Combined with the communication skills in the previous chapter and the mindfulness breathing techniques, you'll have a constructive way of expressing how you feel to others without exploding in anger or saying something harmful. When you begin to feel the onset of what you would consider a "negative" emotion, you can use your breath to help you in the moment. I've relied on my breath more times than I can count just to be able to keep it together until I can find the nearest bathroom or rush out to the car and burst into tears of frustration. When I was in company command, my coworkers thought I had allergies since I'd frequently come out of the bathroom with red eyes and a runny nose. We often need a good cry, another way to release toxins from the body – just not in front of the people you work with. So, yeah, I had "allergies."

Accepting your emotions is to be present in the moment. The military tends to frown on the overt showing of emotions for valid reasons. We want our leaders to be in control and not flying off the handle at every hurdle or setback that occurs. We want our service members to be calm in the face of the chaos of war. All the more reason for learning and practicing these mindfulness techniques. We then would have the tools and skills we need to navigate the extreme situations we face in the military. We as humans fail when we try to reach some idealized version (usually dictated by society or the media) of perfection, and then repeatedly beat ourselves up mentally for failing. Society tells us that we can have it all, a successful career, an amazing and happy marriage, a satisfying sex life, healthy and intelligent children, a beautiful home that's organized and clean, and any other number of things that we see in the form of print, television, or social media. What society doesn't tell us is how this is supposed to happen and that to experience and appreciate joy, we also have to experience pain and go through contrast. You cannot have one without the other. If you try to push away what you consider to be "bad" feelings, you'll end up also not fully being able to feel the "good" feelings. No person is always happy all the time; I don't care what you think you are seeing on social media. You are never alone, whether it's in joy and love, or pain and loss.

If you're uncomfortable attending a group yoga class, or what is available to you doesn't work in your schedule, I recommend yogatoday. com for beginners and all levels. They have a free trial offer and many different styles of yoga you can try. The key is to try yoga and meditation and stay with it, practicing at least once a week for six to eight weeks. Yoga produces results in a subtle and gradual manner. It requires just as much commitment and discipline as you would apply to any exercise program.

# CHAPTER 6

# Develop Your Mindset

*"We are entering the dimension where we
have control – the inside."*
– *Loving What Is*, Byron Katie

By far the greatest amount of growth I have experienced has been in the area of mindset. Flying First-Class is essentially all about mindset. You have the ability to feel the way you want to feel without the condition actually existing. Have you ever been excited about taking a vacation or an upcoming holiday? You felt excitement *before* you actually took the vacation or the holiday occurred. Thus, you had the feeling in advance of the event. I've found that our mindset influences every other aspect of our lives and sets the foundation for all the other skills and strategies in this book. Mindset is that important. Without a healthy mindset, it is virtually impossible to achieve that which we desire. Thinking positive seems like a simple enough task, but mindset is more than just thinking positive. We have to be aware enough of our thoughts in the first place before we can change the way that we think or what thoughts we choose to continue thinking.

I used to think that I hated people. "I hate people," would be a thought I would say to myself daily and out loud to my friends. I thought people were generally stupid and did things to annoy me on purpose. Never mind that this is a self-centered way to view the world, it also guarantees that I will in fact attract people that do what I consider to be stupid things just to annoy me. You may already be familiar with the concept of "The Law of Attraction," which is essentially that we reap what we sow. If you're able to look back objectively at the events and situations in your life, you may be able to see patterns of repetition and remember your mindset during that time.

For example, in my career I went through a six-year period where I had a series of bad bosses, seven to be exact. They kept getting worse and I could not figure out what was going on. I knew enough about Law of Attraction to understand that I had something to do with it, but I had no idea that my continued focus on how awful I perceived these people to be as leaders was essentially continuing the cycle. You may think that it's just a coincidence that I had seven bad leaders in a row, but I do not believe in coincidences. Similar situations show up repeatedly in our lives until we figure out the lesson. In my case, I did not figure it out. I continued to focus on the bad leadership and blame an entire career field that I believed to be full of incompetent leaders. I know now this is not the case. I attracted these leaders because I believed all of them to be bad. The universe simply shows us what we expect to see. After the first bad leader, I expected to see more and I definitely got what I expected. I was looking for the negative. It never occurred to me to look for the positive attributes in these leaders. It wasn't until I was assigned to a unit and job out of my career field that everything changed. I can look back now with 20/20 hindsight and see that because I was going to work in a completely different field, I expected the leaders and the work to be better. Sure enough, it was. Yet again, I got what I expected. Only after I received the mindset training was I able to piece the puzzle together.

Our attitudes have a major effect on what shows up in our lives. If we continually put out judgment and negativity toward other people, we will continue to get all of that back. In my personal journey, I have identified a sure-fire path to my insecurity and it has to do with what I call the three Cs: Compare, Control, and Compete. When

I find that I am comparing my accomplishments to those of others, I inevitably feel that I am inadequate and not adding up. Olivia Fox Cabane says in her book *The Charisma Myth*, "The very act of comparing and evaluating hinders our ability to be fully present." How can I be focusing on what I need to do in this moment if I'm constantly worried about what others are doing? I can't. The same is true when I try to control others. The only person we can ever control is ourselves. Trying to control someone else uses up valuable energy that we do not get back. Byron Katie, in her book *Loving What Is*, mentions three types of business: "God's business, other people's business, and your business." If we are worrying about the first two, then we're not in our own business. Who's minding our business if we're focused on the first two? No one, and we are not fully present in the moment. Plus, when we inevitably realize that we cannot control our husband, children, friends, etc., we experience suffering at our perceived failure or lack of progress in getting what we want. This is because what we want, control of others, is the wrong thing to focus on.

The final C, compete, is harder to eradicate in a military environment. Well, all three Cs are difficult to eliminate in a military environment, since the military thrives on competition, comparison, and control. However, I'm suggesting a healthier relationship to the three Cs by eliminating thought patterns that take us out of our own business. There is always going to be competition within a military environment. We're competing in friendly athletic or military events. We compete for the best evaluations and key positions. However, if we allow the competitive environment to constantly occupy our minds, we'll be missing valuable opportunities to connect with ourselves and other people. Instead of focusing on competition, I chose to focus on collaboration. By collaborating and focusing on the team environment, we could accomplish the mission that much faster and improve the overall unit communication and staff processes. This is a much better and easier mental space from which to operate on a day-to-day basis. Of course, only one officer or enlisted service member can ultimately be number one, but what you accomplish together is far more important than who gets the top place. After all, we volunteered to join the military not because we wanted to be famous and number one. The military is the wrong career choice for fame and fortune. We joined because we wanted to serve in some capacity and service means working with and collaborating with others.

Mindset is a change in perception coupled with a change in attitude. Consider the story of a former coworker of mine who believed that he was not qualified to do his job and that people thought he was stupid. I knew this to be untrue, but what continued to show up for him, under-performance in his evaluations both written and oral, facilitated his belief that he was lacking the skills needed to do the work. We proceeded to have several mindset discussions, and on the sur-face, changing one's mindset seems like it could be an easy thing to do. However, rooted patterns of negative thinking can be difficult to unset. We must first become aware of our thoughts and then choose to stop focusing on the thoughts that do not serve us. My coworker's continued focus on his perceived lack of ability led to fear about per-forming any tasks. Making decisions out of fear or trying to do anything from within that mindset is a real difficult place to be and leads to despera-tion. Rarely does anything good come from a des-perate act. We first had to work on recognizing the negative thoughts and stopping them before they spiraled out of control. I recommended medita-tion, which my coworker responded to with much trepidation and eye-rolling, though he was willing to try. Again, a meditation session can be as short as two minutes and still have the intended results of noticing the thoughts and focusing the mind's attention on a singularity. Next, we had to focus the mind on thoughts that would better serve him to accomplish his goals of performing better and succeeding in his job.

Now, here we come to the tricky part. Focusing on better thoughts alone often does not do the trick to achieving success. Remember how the mind and body are connected? This means that the two must work in harmony for us to achieve physical, mental, and emotional well-being. So not only do we need to think better thoughts, we also need to feel as if what we want to accomplish has already occurred in the present moment. You may be asking yourself, how the heck can I do this? Well, think back to the vacation and holiday example from the beginning of the chapter. Or, maybe it was a birth-day party – but remember the last time you were super excited about something. In most cases, we feel excitement leading up to the event before the event has even occurred. We can feel excitement, happiness, and joy before we've even done the activity because we know the activity is going to happen soon. The same can be true when we're working to change our mindset. We can choose to think better and have focused thoughts (on what we do want versus what we don't want and what we do not have) and we can choose to feel like we would feel if what we want were already true. By bringing the mind (thoughts) and body (emotions) together, we're likely to have more success achieving what we want.

Guided meditations that concentrate on thoughts, feelings, and sensation in the body help us to practice this muscle of combining thoughts and emotions to achieve our goals. Traditional yoga nidra and iRest yoga nidra (secularized yoga nidra) are two forms of meditation that focus on awareness of thoughts, sensation in the body, and emotions, giving people the ability to transcend or move forward without dissociating from thoughts and emotions we perceive as negative or traumatic. I suggested to my coworker that he try iRest meditations, which you can find for free on iRest.us and exaltedwarrior.com. Over the course of a few weeks, he became more conscious of his thoughts, stopped the negative thinking, and switched to thinking about what he did want and feeling how he would feel upon achieving that which he wanted. This practice takes discipline, as we are changing the way we think and have probably thought in default mode for our entire life. His performance at work began to improve. His bosses began to notice the improvement and praise him for his efforts. He felt more confident and continued to believe that he would succeed. When it became time for him to relocate to his next duty station, he was one of the top performers in his section and his superiors could see the vast improvements that he had made in his work. This all started with him choosing to believe, focus, and feel things being better even though the conditions did not exist initially.

These mindset skills aren't just for adults. I've used them successfully with my children. Kamron had a soccer tryout coming up about which he was extremely nervous. Like most humans, his mind immediately went to, "What if I don't make the team?" Here he was focusing and putting all his precious mental energy on exactly what he didn't want to happen. I asked him what did he want. He said he wanted to make the team. I asked him how he would feel once he made the team. He said happy and grateful. I then told him to imagine himself making the team and, most importantly, to feel in his body happy and grateful. Being a dutiful child, he did what I asked in the days leading up to the tryouts. He made the team. When I asked him how he felt, he said happy and grateful. Now, Thomas and I had been working with him months prior with his fitness and soccer drills. However, Kamron can easily put himself into a doom and gloom mindset and let his nerves get the best of him. The mindset training helped in this case. He went on to notice the difference in how his mindset affected his play during games. After a particularly tough loss in which he blamed himself and poor defense for the team losing, I asked him what he was thinking when a player was coming at him with the ball. He said he was thinking, "I don't want to make a mistake." Guess what happened? He made lots of mistakes, since he was thinking about mistakes. I told him to instead think something like, "I steal the ball, I pass the ball, we own the ball," thus focusing his thoughts and energy on action for the team's defense. The change in his demeanor and play the very next game was remarkable. "Who is this kid?" I thought to myself. We're still working on mindset, but imagine the rock stars your kids will be if they learn this at such a young age!

A simple way to put yourself in a better feeling state and raise your energy level is to practice a daily attitude of gratitude. Upon waking each morning, mentally list all the things for which you are grateful and notice how it feels in your body to be grateful. Combining grateful thoughts with feeling grateful in your body will put you in a higher energy state as you go about your day. Coming from a place of gratitude, compassion, and kindness impacts us greatly when making decisions in our lives, from something as simple as choosing to let a vehicle go in front of us, to more complicated choices like deciding on a career, school, or life partner. Making a decision from a place of fear, anger, or desperation always results in hardship or misery in the long run. But how do we know our emotional state when we're making decisions?

Along with using the tools in this book to become more self-aware of our thoughts and emotions, I've developed an acronym that I use when making decisions big or small. SAGE stands for Spacious, Abundant, Grateful, and Easeful. "Sage" also means wisdom, and that was definitely by design. Before making a decision, ask yourself the following: Will whatever it is make me feel Spacious, Abundant, Grateful, and Easeful? Here's an example from my own life. Kamron wanted badly to be in Scouts. I held off for a long time because with my husband in Battalion Command, I knew the responsibility would fall solely on me. Plus, Cub Scouts relies heavily on the mothers. The questions looked something like this. Will being a Den Mother make me feel *spacious* in my schedule physically and mentally? In other words, did I really have enough time to dedicate to being at all the meetings and the prep beforehand? Heck no. The last thing I wanted to do was let my son down. Will being a Den Mother make me feel *abundant* in my life? Will I feel as if the time and commitment I put out will bring to me so much more in return with regards to my son and the other children I can potentially help? Probably not, since I already felt I had a lack of time – this would've added to my stress. Will being a Den Mother make me feel *grateful*? Will this feel like a blessing or a chore of obligation, which could lead to a feeling of resentment? Obligation, for sure at that point in time. Will being a Den Mother make me feel *easeful*? Will it be appropriately challenging but not arduous or forced? Will I have the resources I need or know where to get them? I'm sure I could've figured it out, but the *spacious, abundant,* and *grateful* answers were leaning me toward a hard no. We didn't write off Scouts for good. Once Kamron was eleven, he joined Boy Scouts and is now well on his way to making Eagle Scout. The questions are to help with a decision for a specific point in time and the answers may change as your situation changes.

In answering the questions, pay attention to how you feel and be honest with yourself. Just because something is a good deed does not mean that you are the person who has to do it all the time. It is better to go through this process and realize that you have to say no upfront than to not ask the questions, become overwhelmed, and have to back out at a later date. I have done the latter so many times and it feels absolutely awful to renege on a commitment because I'm at my wit's end. I've made myself physically ill trying to do too many things because I didn't want to say no or didn't have these questions to ask myself to ensure I can really commit to an obligation. Using SAGE to help you make decisions from a place of compassion and kindness will ensure that you're in the right mindset to live a First-Class Lifestyle.

Mindset is not something that you can master within a few weeks or even a lifetime. You can, however, use the tools in this chapter and the MINDFULL Way to begin your journey. Here I will say that it helps immensely to have a coach and a community to bring your attention back to where it needs to be. If you're new in observing and becoming aware of your thoughts, it's often difficult to recognize that you're falling back into a thought pattern that does not serve you. We always rise higher with a community or tribe behind us than we do by ourselves. Find your tribe and change your mindset.

CHAPTER 7

# Find Your Power

In addition to having a focused and positive mindset, identifying and harnessing your internal power source is essential to living a First-Class Lifestyle. Too often, we attach our self-worth to external conditions or people. If the conditions cease to exist or the person fails us in some way, our self-esteem plummets because we have latched on to an external source of power. I realized, upon retirement, that I had quite a bit of my identity wrapped up in being a lieutenant colonel in the Army. Wearing the uniform and commanding the respect of my rank held a lot of power for me. Power in that I felt I belonged, I mattered, and I was secure in my place in the world. I wanted to retire from the Army. I was ready. However, a few months later, I found myself in a funk that I could not explain. I certainly did not want to be on active duty again, but after much journaling and self-reflection, I understood that the uniform and all it symbolizes for me had been my external source of power.

When I put on the uniform, I felt I had authority, protection, confidence, respect, and strength. The uniform also hid my body and essentially masked my femininity and sexuality, which made it easier to downplay those characteristics while at work. In my lieutenant and captain days, the uniform helped me be androgynous, making it easier for me to lead and work with men. Later, I began to become okay with showing more femininity, but I still had the cut of the uniform to hide and protect me. Once that was gone, I had to wear regular clothes. I didn't know who I was or who to be and it was unsettling. It wasn't until I put on a pair of hiking boots to go for a walk that I had my "a-ha" moment. I missed my boots! I missed how I felt in the Army Combat Uniform. How could clothing make me feel powerful? It symbolized something greater to which I no longer belonged – the active duty military community.

Now I had to find an internal source for all those aspects of power that the uniform represented for me. Unconsciously, I had tried to make being an entrepreneur and starting a business fill that external power void. However, no matter how much action I took or how many projects I started, I still felt unfulfilled. I had to first understand that I had attached my self-worth to an external source and identify it, and then I could go about substituting internal sources. This isn't always an easy thing to recognize. Had it not been for the self-awareness tools I've laid out in the previous chapters, I might still be in a place of confusion, heading toward depression.

## Identify External Power Sources

Get honest and real with yourself. The self-communication exercises of the inner dialogue and morning pages are key here. What, if it were to disappear tomorrow, would take your self-worth along with it? The answer could be a person, an object, a career, a company, virtually anything. Whatever it is (it could be multiple things), it allows you to feel safe, like you belong, and like you matter. We all to some degree have external sources of power. It's natural to have them. Often it's our career and our children. If we've done well at work, passed a difficult exam, or received a good evaluation, we feel good about ourselves. If we bombed a briefing, missed a suspense, or failed the height-weight, we feel like crap. Similarly, if our children behave, do well in school, have lots of friends, and are good at sports, music, or some other extracurricular activity, we feel pride and that we're doing a good job. But what happens if they are struggling in one of these areas? Do we blame ourselves, our parenting skills, our absence due to deployments or TDYs? Do we now feel guilt and that we are less than the mother next door who stays home with her children? I did. These are external sources of power. They only become a problem if they are our only source of power because they are not eternal and not within our control. Attaching your self-worth to a person, object, or condition outside yourself sets you up for repeated disappointment and a self-esteem roll-ercoaster ride. If you're worried about what your mother, boss, husband, or friends think of you and that determines your mood for the day, then you've given them power and control over you. Of course, to some degree, we care about what others think, or we wouldn't be able to live in society and conform to military standards. What determines whether or not you have an unhealthy attachment to an exter-nal source for your power is how you respond when circumstances remove the source. As was the case with me, I felt lost for a good several months after retirement, before I realized what was going on. A friend of mine was told by her peers that she was no longer useful to the unit after she had become pregnant. The male officers now had to cover for her because she could no longer carry a weapon and ride in a HMMWV. How do you think that made her feel? Not cool, and resentful toward them and the military. This happened well before 2008 and I did not have the skills to offer any words of advice. I PCS'd soon after. My point is that relying solely on what others think can lead to unnecessary shame and despair. Who are they to tell us we are not useful? We're creating a human being inside of our bodies! It's likely the most useful and important thing we will ever do! After identifying the source, you now have to determine what characteristics it represents for you. Does the external source symbolize wealth, status, confidence, sexuality, freedom, vitality, youth, acceptance? These are just a few examples out of dozens or hundreds of symbols for your power source.

## Replacing Symbols with Internal Sources

Reclaiming your power from external sources means you have to determine how you can bridge the gap to make symbols from the external source of power something that you are able to generate internally. Let me explain further using my own example of the uniform. For each characteristic or role the uniform played for me, I identified another characteristic that I would always have because I create it internally and I define it.

The Uniform as:

- **Authority** – became my sense of Purpose. Certainly my purpose can change, but it is always something that I create, I define, and I can have several. My purpose is to share my story and what I've learned with you so that I can help others. My purpose is to bring mindfulness, meditation, and yoga to the military so that I can help others. My purpose is to raise two children to be healthy and productive members of society. My purpose gives me that sense of authority and direction I had while in the military.

- **Protection** – became my Spirituality. My faith in a God and a Universe that has my back and is working in my favor provides me a much stronger protection than the uniform or the Army ever did. No one can take away my faith or spirituality. I alone choose what I believe.

- **Confidence** – became my Love of Self. I know I am a good person doing the best that I can do. Sure, I make mistakes, but my intent is coming from a place of kindness, love, and compassion. My confidence comes from being okay with who I am in each moment (a benefit of consistent meditation) and all parts of me, light and shadow.

- **Respect** – became my Choice to Help Others. I craved respect. Without the uniform, no one knew who I was or what I had done. This bothered me in a big way. I had a choice – we always have choices; I could continue to lament about people not knowing I had ever served in the military, or I could continue to serve and help others, creating my own self-respect for me. I cannot force other people to respect me. If they choose to respect me because of my work and achievements, that is fantastic. I needed to respect myself and the way for me to do that was to help others any way I could.

- **Strength** – became Valuing my Experiences and Knowledge. As I mentioned earlier in this book, I am prone to undervaluing myself. This is a huge problem and robs me of a fantastic source of strength. I asked you earlier to list your accomplishments so you can appreciate all you've done. Theoretically, someone could take away some of your accomplishments. For example, the Army could say they miscalculated the dates and that I hadn't served enough time to retire. That would really suck and is why my source of strength does not rely solely on accomplishments. The Army cannot take away the experiences I've had while serving and the knowledge I've gained. This gives me strength, and every day I have new experiences and gain more knowledge, thus continuously renewing my source of strength.

- **Masked Femininity** – became my connection to Mind, Body, and Soul. Masking my femininity wasn't a good thing for me to do all those years, but it's what I felt I had to do to lead effectively. I was confusing femininity with sexuality and did not want that in the workplace. I realized I was wrong through the help of a life coach and started to reacquaint myself with my feminine side toward the latter part of my career. However, the feeling of being naked in regular clothes was still there. A year or so before I retired, a friend convinced me to be in a local pageant. Oh the horror! Do you know what freaked me out the most? It was not having to answer an on-stage question, give an interview, or dance in an opening number. I was most afraid of having to walk across the stage in an evening gown. The judges (unknown to us until the day of the pageant) were members of the local community and I imagined that all of them would be my current bosses – this was my nightmare. Clearly, I still had work to do in the area of reclaiming my femininity. I did the pageant and came in third and faced the seemingly ridiculous fear of wearing a dress. Reconnecting my mind, body, and soul through meditation and yoga helps me to stay whole and appreciate the duality of both my masculine and feminine qualities working equally together.

In order to be successful, you need internal power. Identifying and disconnecting from external sources is the first step toward creating internal power. It's not always easy or comfortable, but is definitely necessary to live a First-Class Lifestyle. It can also be difficult to do alone, and I do recommend a life coach or objective friend that can ask tough questions and see what you maybe cannot.

# CHAPTER 8

# Unleash Your Trust

*"Trust in the LORD with all your heart
and lean not on your own understanding."*
– Proverbs 3:5

A few months ago, I was walking my dog one afternoon and we came upon some ducks floating in a creek. As we walked closer the ducks, who moments before had been effortlessly moving downstream with the current of the creek, turned around and began furiously paddling upstream to try and get away from us. I saw a physical representation of what it's like to paddle upstream, using a whole lot of energy and getting nowhere. The ducks remained in the exact same spot as we got closer. They eventually just got out of the water and ran away from us, but the image stuck in my mind. We as people exert a lot of our precious energy trying to control or force things to go our way when the majority of the time whatever we're trying to make happen is not under our control. We essentially paddle upstream like the ducks and get nowhere. Where, if we were to let go of the oars and allow the current of life to carry us downstream, we would only have to steer and course correct in the form of a focused, positive, and strong mindset. It's a lot easier said than done, yet we trust people every day. On our First-Class flight, we trust the pilots to get us to our destination safely. We trust childcare providers, teachers, coworkers, the mailman to deliver the mail. We have the ability to trust. But trust (with a little "t") is not quite the same as Trust with a big "T."

I'm talking about faith or big Trust in God and a Universe that is on your side and working for your benefit. I first began to really understand and work with the concept of big Trust only after working with my life coach, Kris. It never before occurred to me that I didn't have to be in a continuous state of struggle to get what I wanted. I was always worrying about something and what I needed to do when in fact I just needed to relax. Too often we feel as if the world or certain people are out to get us. However, we've learned in the previous chapters that our thoughts and mindset have a great deal to do with what shows up in our lives. We are energetic beings and if you think of our energy like a radio signal broadcasting out into the world, we will get back that which we put out. The Universe doesn't judge, it just shows us what we expect to see. If we Trust that the Universe is on our team and believe things are always working for our ultimate benefit, we'll begin to notice all the synchronicities that happen in our lives. For example, when I started saying to myself, "I'm always in the right place at the right time, and I always get exactly what I need" (not what I may want), things just started getting done. My unit had decided to make me the "cyber planner." It didn't matter that I am not technical and really don't understand anything about cyber, the previous job I had managing people in that field seemed to be enough credibility. Well, I was not pleased and was terrified everyone would figure out that I had no idea what I was doing. But being that I was working with Kris at the time, I did not focus my thoughts on impending disaster but instead Trusted that things would work out somehow. This was not easy for me to do, but I'd already learned that worrying was just a waste of my precious energy and a form of negative prayer. The newly-formed Cyber Command sent an officer to help my unit build its cyber program. Yes! This guy knew what he was doing and developed and implemented a program that I was able to use successfully until I thankfully deployed and didn't have to do cyber anymore. Things worked out because I Trusted and felt grateful in advance that they would. I learned just enough to stay afloat until the situation changed. I have dozens of these types of examples that are all little things on the surface, but happen so often now as compared to before I focused on Trust. They may seem like coincidences, but I do not believe in coincidence. When things go our way, it's because we are in alignment with our true divine nature, God, Source, the Universe, whatever you choose to call this phenomenon. We fall into alignment by learning to have big Trust. I notice that when I'm trying to force an outcome, I feel tight in my upper back and shoulders and I start holding my breath. However, if I'm in a state of alignment, I feel calm and the task seems effortless. Many coaches and spiritual teachers call this the act of surrendering. This isn't a military-friendly term so if it doesn't feel right, then don't "surrender." You can "let go," "let go of the oars," "relax," "rest" in the palm of God's hand or that of a Higher Power. The point is to remember that we can only control our own thoughts, actions, behavior, and breath. Everything else is not within our personal control and should not be our concern. It's awful stressful to put other people's lives on your shoulders. I am not solely responsible for the well-being of my family, friends, and coworkers. I control my own business.

I believe that they will control their own business and Trust that God has the rest under control. This is especially true as children get older. We nurture them, guide them, teach them about healthy decision-making, but ultimately they have to learn to make their own choices and be responsible for living with the consequences of their actions.

Big Trust is not about religion, but it is spiritual in the belief that humans have souls and are connected to a greater universal consciousness. If this doesn't sit well with you, then I suggest you inquire as to why through some journaling or talking with a close friend that won't judge you for your beliefs. The end goal is not getting you to believe something you don't want to believe, but providing a safe space for you to inquire about your current beliefs and if they are in some way preventing you from experiencing the peace of a First-Class Lifestyle that you deserve in your life. Big Trust isn't an easy concept to swallow for a lot of people. I still have moments of, "Why is this happening to me" instead of, "How is this experience for my ultimate benefit?" This type of thinking requires an entire shift in perspective, which requires you to step outside the situation and observe from the place of a compassionate witness. Once again, a consistent yoga and meditation practice will give you the tools to do this.

The practice of yoga on the mat, how we behave in different postures, often mirrors what we encounter in real life. I have a fear of going upside down. I really am quite terrified to try and do a handstand or a headstand. I am tentative to try up against a wall, but refuse to try in the middle of the room with no support around me. Why? I don't trust myself not to fall. I have in fact fallen trying to do a headstand without a wall. It's frightening and I have fear and hesitation that turns into straight out panic as I topple over. I'm not breathing and my muscles are clenching for dear life. Do I have big Trust issues in real life? You bet. With big life changes, I often don't Trust that I will succeed. Why? I don't know. This is the inquiry that I take to the mat. As I'm writing this, I'm having an "a-ha" moment. I've been resistant to get on my mat daily. I've just figured out why. My practice has been boring and routine because I've been doing the same comfortable and familiar postures for the last several years. I've refused to try anything challenging and definitely not an inversion. Deep down I know that overcoming fear, having faith, big Trust, in my life starts with facing the poses that I fear on the mat. Through experimenting with the dreaded inversions and all the work to strengthen my body to do them safely, I overcome adversity and learn to have big Trust that I will acquire the abilities and skills I need to achieve the task. Crap. I'm afraid and that's why I've been avoiding my yoga practice. When we notice ourselves being continuously resistant to someone or something, this is the time for self-inquiry. Usually, the resistance involves a fear. By working through the fear or adversity, we strengthen our faith and unleash big Trust. As you see, this is not something you can master by the end of this book or even in a lifetime. We are continually learning and experiencing how to Trust.

## CHAPTER 9

# Lighten Your Shadow

*"The highest spiritual practice is self-observation without judgment."*
– Swami Kripalu

Now we come to the most difficult chapter for me to write: the chapter on self-sabotage and obstacles that can prevent you from having the First-Class Lifestyle you desire and deserve. It's difficult for me in that I struggle with how much of my personal experience to share. Dealing with our shadow side is not always easy and generally we tend to ignore or run away from those parts of ourselves that we do not like. The thing about shadows though, they are connected to you always. You cannot outrun your shadow. What do I mean by your shadow side? This is the side of you that has thoughts you wouldn't dare tell another soul and may not even want to write down for fear of admitting they exist. This is the side of you that society says is bad and most easily relates to the seven deadly sins of anything that is prideful, greedy, lustful, envious, gluttonous, wrathful, or slothful. I absolutely have thoughts like these.

Here's what you need to know. Having these types of thoughts is completely normal and now that you know how to be aware of them through meditation and yoga, you have the mindset tools to deal with them. We don't need to act on these thoughts and we also don't need to lament over the fact that they exist. We do, however, need to accept this shadow side as a part of who we are, whether we like it or not. For when we don't and we try to ignore this part of ourselves or run away, that's when we start seeing the same difficult situations come up repeatedly. Remember my story of the series of bad bosses? This contrast kept showing up in my life. What part of myself was I not acknowledging? From what was I running? Turns out I place judgment on people like a champ. I am so quick to pass judgment and yet ignore the very same trait within myself. These bosses were a mirror reflecting my secret feelings and projections of insecurity, incompetence, dislike of people, and judgment. It took hindsight to see all this and accept the fact that I have the shadow side of confidence, competence, love of people, and compassion.

The shadow side will usually have something to do with an unhealthy relationship to one of the three Cs – control, compete, compare. I notice jealousy comes up when I continuously compare myself to other people. This can become insidious without you even realizing. My house was never as neat or clean as my neighbor's house. How could it be? I was working full time and didn't have a cleaning lady. I didn't bake as well as the woman down the street. Probably because I don't enjoy baking. Yet this logic gets lost in the self-sabotaging act of comparison, which leads to jealousy. And there I went again, spiraling into a pit of despair. I would never be enough if I continued to compare my weaknesses to other people's strengths. I had to learn to accept myself as I was and praise my accomplishments, not continually highlight my weaknesses. I also learned to transform jealousy into genuine admiration for people's talents and skills. This is a mindset shift, a change in perception.

I used to have an unhealthy competitive attitude when it came to attending yoga class. I was secretly competing with the other yogis in the class. I was always looking around, comparing yet again, and lamenting that my poses didn't look as good or I wasn't as flexible. It got so bad that I had to stop going to class. I had sabotaged my own yoga practice. These are characteristics of ourselves that are normal, but don't have to control us if we become aware of them and face them head on. When I stopped ignoring these aspects of myself and shined some light on them, I realized that I did not need to be afraid of myself, other people, or periods of adversity. The contrast happens so that I may learn something and grow from the experience. The fear of failing as a mother and at my job were real. I looked for blame everywhere else rather than looking inside and facing those fears. Facing those fears would mean having to accept them and the fact that I physically could not survive trying to do everything by myself. My pride and ego demanded that I show everyone I could do it alone, but I was drowning in pride and ego, and the fear of admitting that I was wrong and asking people for help almost made me fail for real. Some of my other challenges have been even more painful than that time at West Point and involve loved ones, but we all have them and you are not alone. Through using the tools of yoga, meditation, and life coaches, I was able to recognize, accept, and honor all parts of who I am. It takes yet more discipline to not run away when faced with emotional fear. These fears felt just as real as if I had come across a stranger with a knife in a dark alley. They were dark places in the far corners of my mind, mainly because I had pushed them there and refused to confront them. Yoga and meditation helped me to understand that fear, like other emotions, does not stay forever. It's fluid and can move on as quickly as it came. Fear has played an important role in the evolution of the human race, preventing us from harming ourselves or putting ourselves in dangerous situations. Fear is a companion and as physical dangers became less frequent as humans evolved, we began to look at fear as a sign of weakness. Fear is not a weakness, it's a tool. Fear shines light on areas that need our attention for our overall expansion and growth. Fear is a friend and understanding how to work with fear will make you more powerful than you can ever be by ignoring it.

Maybe your shadow side has to do with control and your need to always be in charge. I had a friend who was like this. Whether it's something like consistently dominating the conversation, telling me how he thinks I should feel in a situation, or never asking for my opinion, his need to be in control sabotaged our friendship. What was he afraid of? I don't know. I don't know what you're afraid of either, only that you have fears. I do know that the characteristics that bother you about other people often are the same shadow characteristics in yourself. I didn't want this friend to try and control me, yet at home I was trying to control Thomas,

Kamron, and Violette. My daughter in particular has shown me that this will not work. She gets angry, wild, and sometimes vicious. The more I tried to control her and make her do my will, the more she resisted. When we went to the child psychologist to help with her anger management, I realized that me always needing to be in control over her was the equivalent of me micromanaging one of my subordinates. I would never do that to someone at work. I prided myself on empowering my subordinates. But with my daughter, I felt she needed to do what I told her. I'm the parent, after all. The situation doesn't exactly correlate to work because she is a minor child and I am legally responsible for her, but empowering her to take control of her emotions with the tools she learned from therapy was a step in the right direction.

Take some time to objectively look back at situations in your life where you felt afraid and notice if any of them are reoccurring. Do you notice the same type of irritating person time and time again? Or maybe you always find yourself in the role of the victim? How did you react or handle each situation? The victim role is something I see over and over again in coworkers and friends. The situations they find themselves in always seem to be somebody else's fault and have nothing to do with their own actions. Unfortunately, we can't rescue them.

I've tried. In my early days on this self-aware-ness journey, I just loved to tell people what was wrong with them and give them my good unso-licited advice. This was not helpful. You cannot change anyone but yourself. If you use the tools of awareness in this book, you'll be able to recognize situations that repeat and the underlying fear asso-ciated with those situations. This is where the trans-formation happens, through the fear, contrast, and adversity. Understanding what you are afraid of can help you confront future situations from a place of compassion for and acceptance of yourself. In fact, once you confront the fear, you may not have any more situations that present the fear to you. How-ever, life will always bring you something to deal with at some point. Meditation, yoga, journaling, and self-reflection will help you stay vigilant.

## CHAPTER 10

# Live and Maintain

Now that you know how you can have a First-Class Lifestyle, it's important to also know what to do to maintain that lifestyle. This is perhaps the step that so many people either skip over or forget. Just like with physical fitness, if you don't maintain some sort of regular practice, your emotional and mental fitness will decline. You will always come up against contrast as an opportunity for continued growth and expansion. There's no way out of it as long as you are alive. Use the resources available to you to help you stay organized and manage your time efficiently. Accept the fact that you cannot do everything on your own and reach out for help. It is not a sign of weakness, I promise you. Continue to work on your communication skills to improve your relationship not only with yourself, but with your partner, family, friends, coworkers, and all the other people in your life. Just because I've written this book doesn't mean that I've arrived anywhere or that my learning and growing are done. We may be in different life stages or have different skills, but we're always continuing to progress and move forward. It's also important to not compare your step one to someone else's step twenty.

Develop some sort of physical and emotional practice (I like yoga and meditation) to observe, feel, and process your emotions. This will also help you to become more aware of your thoughts and give you the ability to manage your mindset that much better. Identify external power sources and how you can disconnect from them in favor of an internal power source. Know that you are not alone and Trust that the Universe is on your team and working in your favor. Learn to become aware of your shadow and shine the light of awareness on your fears so that you can transform through them.

Finally, maintain all of these skills through regular self-care, i.e. go on vacation, a retreat, or just take a break. The body and the mind need rest. The military seems to be anti-rest, but is making great strides with mindfulness programs at Army Wellness Centers, Resiliency Training, and working with non-profit organizations like Warriors at Ease. There is no solution more perfect to taking a break from a busy life than just "not doing" and allowing the body and mind to do nothing or "no-thing."

Regular meditative practices like yoga nidra or iRest allow the mind and body to rest and recharge. Going on vacation (and *not* trying to see and do everything) or taking a retreat designed for self-care are also important. You deserve to spend your hard-earned money on your well-being. Being in the military and a mother, everybody needs something from you and it usually feels like they need it immediately. Your nature may be to put everyone else's needs before your own. This is not a sustainable way of living and will lead to your burnout and resentment of the very people that genuinely need your care. You are being selfish in a good way when you do take the time to put yourself first for a few minutes a day, an hour or two a week, one day a month, and one or two weeks out of the year. Self-care looks like the following for me: Daily – yoga (time varies depending on the day, but as little as fifteen minutes is still beneficial), twenty to thirty minutes for meditation and walking; Weekly – two to four hours of alone time to read, hike, or explore a new place; Yearly – some sort of yoga retreat, training, or vacation by myself. Taking the time to schedule your self-care will make all the difference in your ability to maintain a First-Class Lifestyle. I continue to work regularly with my mentors and coaches. Remember that you are not alone in your struggle. I've been in your shoes and

I'm here to support you. Your family and friends will support you if you ask them. Life isn't meant to always be easy, but it's a lot more enjoyable with the help of others and the mindset that you can feel like you're flying First-Class no matter what the circumstances.

# Acknowledgments

This book is a result of all the cumulative lessons I've learned from every single person I've ever met. As it would be impossible to list each individual by name, the highlights include all my yoga, meditation, mindfulness, mindset, and life coaches (whether you knew it or not): Seane, Joyce, Caroline, Brahmani, Jashoda, Kris, Wayne, Meredith, Vanessa, Jen, and Angela.

My support network of family and friends who believed in me when I did not, but especially Thomas, Shay, Megan, Mom, and Dad.

To the Morgan James Publishing team: Special thanks to David Hancock, CEO & Founder for believing in me and my message. To my Author Relations Manager, Gayle West, thanks for making the process seamless and easy. Many more thanks to everyone else, but especially Jim Howard, Bethany Marshall, and Nickcole Watkins.

And of course, all the Soldiers, NCOs, officers, service members, civilians, and contractors I've ever worked with and for. Without you (SFC Soto, 1SG Von, the Army Red Team, SGM Sutton, and so many more), I would never have grown into a leader or known how to take care of people. You're the reason I stayed in for twenty and the reason I went to work each morning. If not for you, I would've quit a long time ago. Thank you for encouraging me and being there for me.

# About the Author

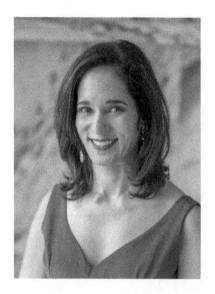

Benef Verell retired from the Army as a lieutenant colonel after serving twenty years on active duty. A West Point graduate, she received her commission in 1997 as a Military Police officer. Later, after getting her master's degree in physical geography and teaching at West Point, she changed her career field to Information Operations.

It was during this time, while teaching at West Point with her husband deployed and two young children, that she began searching for ways to cope with the stress of her job and motherhood. In 2008, Benef attended her first yoga retreat and thus began a lifelong journey towards understanding mindfulness and its benefits on the mind and body.

After her deployment to Iraq in 2012, Benef attended the 200-hour yoga teacher training at the Kripalu Center for Yoga and Health in Stockbridge, Massachusetts. It was here she learned the life-changing skill of being fully present in the moment. She applied this and many other valuable mindfulness tools to her daily life at work and at home. She has helped dozens of friends, coworkers, and family members work through their internal struggles by passing on the knowledge she gained from her personal yoga practice and life coaching.

She's taught private and group yoga and meditation classes on deployments and in military communities since 2013. She's a certified Warriors at Ease yoga instructor and teaches trauma sensitive and adaptive yoga. As a retiree and an Army spouse, Benef continues to volunteer and serve in military communities. She enjoys traveling the world with her husband and two children and living wherever the Army takes them.

# Thank You

L et's keep talking!

Thank you for reading *Military and Mindful*! I sincerely hope this book has provided you with the tools you need to manage your military career along with motherhood. As you develop your skills through the MINDFULL process, you may have questions, challenges, or comments.

Please know that you are not alone.

Reach out to me via email at

benef@militaryandmindful.com

and we can schedule a free strategy session to discuss how I can best serve you. I hope to hear from you soon!

9 781642 794670